Anorexia

A guide to understanding anorexia, improving the condition, and overcoming it

Table Of Contents

Introduction iv
Chapter 1 - Understanding the Totality of
Anorexia 1
Chapter 2 - The Other Side of Anorexia 5
Chapter 3 - Causes Of Anorexia: Who Is
At Risk? 9
Chapter 4 - Determining Anorexia
Through Tests and Diagnostic Exams 13
Chapter 5 - Focus of Treatment For
Anorexia 16
Chapter 6 - Bidding Farewell to Anorexia 20
Conclusion 21

Introduction

I want to thank you and congratulate you for downloading the book, *"Anorexia: A guide to understanding anorexia, improving the condition, and overcoming it"*.

This book contains helpful information about anorexia, and how you can begin to understand, and improve it!

Anorexia has a range of different causes and contributing factors, and there is no simple cure to the condition.

This book will teach you about the signs and symptoms of anorexia, how anorexia is developed, and most importantly how it can be overcome.

You will learn about the different treatments used for anorexia, including medical strategies as well as different types of therapies that can be used.

Overcoming anorexia is not always easy, but if you tackle it as soon as the symptoms begin to become apparent, it's a lot easier to overcome. You will soon discover where to go to help when battling anorexia, and be provided with some simple action steps that you can take.

This book will explain to you tips and techniques that will allow you to successfully understand the condition of anorexia and work on improving it! Whether you personally suffer from anorexia, or you're worried about a family member or friend, this book will have something to offer you.

I wish you the best of luck, and hope this book is able to help you in your journey!

Thanks again for downloading this book, I hope you enjoy it!

Chapter 1 - Understanding the Totality of Anorexia

Food is man's real best friend. You literally cannot live without it. And yet, there are times that you lose the urge to eat. You simply do not have the appetite for food.

There are many possible reasons why a person loses the desire to eat. For instance, when one is too excited or the opposite of that, one is too sad or depressed. In times like these, the inclination to consume food is diminished. When things are back to normal, the regular eating habit is resumed. This is considered as a normal response.

However, there is a medical condition known as anorexia where the lack or loss of appetite for food is not normal anymore.

What is anorexia?

Anorexia, also known as anorexia nervosa, is a potentially life threatening eating disorder that affects mostly young females. Those who are afflicted with this condition are called anorexics. An anorexic can be so engrossed with losing weight that his or her health becomes compromised.

There are two types of Anorexia. The first one is called the restricting type. This is the more common type where the person tries to lose weight by watching thoroughly the calorie count through drastic diet or by exercising too much. The second one is called the purging type. In this type, the anorexic eats, but later on induces vomiting or uses laxatives and diuretics to remove the ingested food.

An anorexic individual usually manifests the following behaviors:

- Has an intense fear of gaining weight even though the current weight is below the normal already
- Is in denial that something is wrong with his or her weight or eating habits
- Has a distorted body image wherein one sees himself or herself as fat when they are actually very thin
- Although there is an aversion to food, an anorexic is very much preoccupied with thoughts of foods and dieting, losing weight, and becoming thin
- Refuses to maintain the ideal body weight

These behaviors can result in physical health complications of the heart, liver, gastrointestinal, kidneys and other vital organs of the body.

Physical effects of Anorexia

Here is the list of what a person may experience physically while suffering from Anorexia.

- Dry skin
- Brittle nails
- Purplish extremities (due to poor tissue perfusion)
- Thinning of hair
- Imbalances in electrolytes and essential minerals
- Tooth decay
- Headaches
- Abdominal pain
- Bruising easily
- Deficiency in iron and zinc
- Appearance of lanugo or fine hairs all over the body, including the face

Other physiological damage may include hormonal disturbances, which can lead to cessation of menstrual periods among girls (this is usually the first sign) and unfortunately sometimes, permanent infertility. The hormonal imbalances may lead to the following:

- Stunting of height and growth due to reduced growth hormones
- Reduced production of estrogen, which is vital to achieving healthy heart and bones
- Increased release and reproduction of stress hormones called cortisol
- Reduced thyroid hormone, which is the one responsible for metabolism, temperature control, growth and development. For infants, thyroid hormone is crucial for the normal development of the brain.
- For males, there is a decreased sex drive or libido and impotence due to low testosterone levels

Take note that other systems of the body may also be affected such as the following:

- Nervous system – affecting the brain functions, memory, decision-making skills and comprehension
- Gastrointestinal system – may lead to ulcers, reflux, constipation, among other things
- Blood problems such as low blood count, poor perfusion
- Skeletal system - reduced bone density (which can lead to osteoporosis and bone fractures)

Due to poor nutrition, the immune system is also highly affected making the anorexics very susceptible to infections and illnesses.

Effects on the heart

Heart failure is usually the cause of death of anorexics. This occurs because of the following effects of anorexia on the heart:

- It causes bradycardia (pulse rate of less than 60 beats per minute)
- Decreased flow of oxygenated blood throughout the body and most especially to the heart and other vital organs
- Low blood pressure
- Abnormal rhythm and poor conduction of electrical impulses of the heart due to electrolyte imbalances
- Reduced size of heart muscles due to malnutrition

In the late stage of anorexia, multi-organ failure is very common. When left untreated, these symptoms may progress in severity and eventually result in death.

Anorexia is multi-faceted

Anorexia runs deep, reaching aspects other than the physical. The food and weight issues are just symptoms of something more complex. Further assessment could lead to the discovery of the following conditions: depression, insecurities, low self-esteem, loneliness, feeling of inadequacy, and pressure to be perfect, to name just a few. To conclude, anorexia also involves the emotional, social, mental and psychological aspects of an individual. These areas will be further discussed in the following chapters.

Is there any hope for anorexics?

There is good news awaiting anorexics. Anorexia can be beaten. An individual can overcome this illness and be free forever from its hold. Anorexia is treatable. One can hope for a full recovery from the condition.

Chapter 2 - The Other Side of Anorexia

Anorexia is a serious medical condition that requires immediate and continuous care. It is a potentially fatal illness.

Important Statistics on Anorexia

Anorexia is ranked as the third most prevalent long-term illness of young people. The average onset or starting age for anorexia is 17. There is a disturbing rise in the number of younger individuals being diagnosed, however. There are reports of 10 year olds being diagnosed with this eating disorder. While commonly perceived as a female-only condition, males are not totally immune to this medical condition either. Around 10% of all anorexics are male.

Statistics report that 20% of anorexics will end up dead if the disorder is not treated properly. With early and appropriate treatment however, the probability of death is reduced to 2-3%. Among young women between the ages of 15-24, anorexia is the most common cause of death.

More to Anorexia than meets the eye

Anorexia, though termed as an eating disorder, is actually deeper than just the lost desire for food, excessive dieting and an unhealthy eating habit.

Many people are misled with the concept that Anorexia is all about food and losing weight. Issues about food and weight are just byproducts of a more complicated medical condition.

Further assessment and studies of anorexics reveals that the root cause of the disorder actually starts from the psychological realm.

Anorexia and the Psychological Aspect of Man

Anorexia is commonly accompanied by depression. But does a person develop Anorexia because he or she is depressed? Or is it the other way around, does one have Anorexia and became depressed as a result? No one can be entirely sure.

One can assume that depression is having an effect on an anorexic person when the following symptoms are noticed:

- Unexplained sadness. Expressions of unhappiness could be very evident. When assessed for the reasons for the sadness, the anorexic will usually fail at identifying the factors that contribute to the feeling of sadness.
- Inability to sleep. Depressed people tend to sleep very little.
- Irritable. Possibly due to inadequate rest and sleep, anorexics are often very cranky, severing relations with others.
- Loss of interest in other activities. The primary focus is on weight loss. All thoughts, energy and activities are geared towards losing weight and not eating food.
- Loss of desire for sexual activities. This could be because of hormonal imbalance and decreased strength and energy.

Many health professionals agree that Anorexia is primarily a psychological concern. Being depressed tops the psychological symptoms of Anorexia. Here are other symptoms that are commonly manifested by anorexics:

- Low self-esteem. Anorexics often feel inferior and constantly search to find approval from other people. They have no faith and belief in themselves. They also

tend to have the feeling of worthlessness. Their poor perception of self makes anorexics shy away from social gatherings. They isolate themselves from the crowd. They also experience difficulties in maintaining relationships.
- Always anxious. Anorexics worry all the time. As the condition advances, the tendency to worry increases. They worry mostly about minor concerns such as calorie count or fluctuating in weight. The major issues, such as declining health are inadvertently left out, however.
- Is in denial. Anorexics think and feel that there is nothing wrong with them. They try to cover up thinness by wearing loose clothing. They pretend to eat when with other people. They also get angry when people try to talk them into eating or when other people express concern over their weight.
- Do not pursue other interests. Anorexics are so preoccupied with food and dieting that they do not have time for other things and hobbies. Most of them however, spend a lot of time exercising. They do rigid exercise mostly on their own and with full concentration, not taking the time to socialize with others. Thoughts of losing weight dominate their thinking and actions.
- Feelings of shame and embarrassment. Anorexics' poor self-image leads them to believe that they cannot do anything right. Losing weight makes them feel in control because for once, they think that they are able to accomplish something specific and right. If they fail in this endeavor, they start to feel inferior again.
- Hopelessness. It's a never-ending cycle for anorexics. They try to lose weight, they feel they are gaining weight and they try to lose weight again.
- Development of self-destructive behaviors. Thoughts of harming oneself are very common among anorexics. With feelings of low self-worth, the anorexics do not value their total wellbeing. Self-

mutilation is a way of coping for them. They also are at high risk of committing suicide. It is very important to note that professional treatment for anorexics at this stage is very vital. Seek professional help even before the symptom of self-harm is manifested. Rehabilitation is oftentimes required to protect the patient and other people from harm.

Effects of Anorexia on Social Life

As the person deteriorates into depression, interpersonal relationships are very much affected. The psychological effects of anorexia can result in the following social dilemmas:

- Isolation – as they tend to shy away from social gatherings, anorexics become more and more withdrawn from other people. They prefer to be alone and away from get-togethers or parties. They also tend to brood and be forlorn most of the time.
- Poor interpersonal relationships – as time goes by, anorexics tend to develop mistrust towards other people, especially those who are expressing concern over their health. They have a false belief that these people are against them, and not with them.
- Becoming secretive. They try to hide their aversion to food, for instance pretending to eat when they are with other people or eating and then vomiting later, when nobody is looking. They also try to hide evidence of poor health through clothes, accessories and makeup. They also tend to lie when directly asked about their food intake.
- Marital relationships can be damaged too due to decreased sexual interest of anorexics. This is brought about by hormonal imbalances due to poor nutrition.

Anorexia can be devastating not only to the sufferer, but also to the patient's family and loved ones. Discover more about anorexia and how to overcome it in the next chapter.

Chapter 3 - Causes Of Anorexia: Who Is At Risk?

Anorexia is a complex medical condition. It's not possible to identify the exact cause of the disorder, as various factors may contribute to the acquisition of the condition. It can be caused by a combination of biological, psychological, emotional, social and environmental influences.

Biological Causes

Some people have an increased predisposition to anorexia because of genetics. Studies show that if there is family member who is afflicted with this condition, the likelihood of another member getting it is 10-20 times more than the general population. It could also be due to the family's genetic tendency or culture of gearing towards perfectionism – a trait very evident among anorexics.

Brain chemical imbalance is also considered as a possible cause of Anorexia. There is an increased production and release of the hormone cortisol. This brain hormone is mostly present during stressful episodes. On the other hand, there is a decreased level of serotonin and norepinephrine. These hormones are the ones responsible for the overall feelings of wellbeing.

Psychological/Emotional Causes

Perfectionism can be traced back to during the growing-up years of anorexics. They usually develop an extreme desire for perfection, which may be caused by strict and over controlling parents or harsh treatment and training. They are also usually overachievers. They try to do above and beyond what is required and expected of them. Outwardly, they may seem as accomplished and successful. However inwardly, they often feel worthless, hopeless and helpless.

Being able to control their weight is a form of having control over their lives. It's where they feel that they can attain perfection. Anorexics often even feel pleasure when hunger pains strike.

Social Causes

Another contributory factor is the influence of family, friends and the society as a whole, to be thin. People who have received criticism regarding their bodies and physical appearance due to weight gain can sometimes resort to extreme dieting, and end up developing anorexia.

There are also activities that require slenderness such as modeling, ballet and some sports. The participants have no choice but to follow the weight requirement to be able to continue with the activity. Initially, this is just to comply with the requirement, but later on, the need to continue with the dieting and losing weight can become an obsession.

Environmental Causes

The media has been widely blamed for the rise in the number of anorexics. Images of thin people, especially of women, are common features in magazines, television and movies. Toys like Barbie and the Disney princesses have also been accused of promoting thinness among young women. Being thin is equated to being beautiful and successful.

Who's At Risk Of Developing Anorexia

> ➢ Young women top the list of those who are high risk of developing this medical condition. Around 80-90% of anorexics are women aged between 15-24. There are

rare occurrences among people 40 years old and above.
- Those with familial tendency and an imbalance in brain chemicals are also susceptible.
- Major life events – important life transitions, such as a new school or work, new home, birth or death of a family member or loved one, and illness, can all trigger the onset of Anorexia. An inability to cope with life's challenges and stresses causes an increased release of cortisol and decreased production of serotonin, leading to the depressed state of the individual.
- Weight changes. Most of the time, the positive comments of other people regarding weight loss motivate a person to lose some more weight. Eventually this may lead to excessive weight loss. On the other hand, negative comments about weight increase can challenge a person to lose the weight, sometimes to the extreme. As the anorexic has the tendency to seek approval from other people, the desire to be thin to please these people is ever present.
- Weight loss as a requirement of work, sports or hobbies. People who face the need to meet weight requirements have a higher tendency to develop anorexia. Again, most of these athletes, artists, dancers, actors or models initially started dieting to maintain the needed weight. Eventually the focus on dieting becomes an obsession, and anorexia is developed.
- Those influenced by Western culture are more prone to Anorexia. This could be attributed to media exposure where thinness is more favored.

There are still instances where some people become anorexics even though they are not high risk of developing the condition.

As with all medical conditions, early detection and treatment yields more positive outcomes. Confirm the presence of

Anorexia through tests and diagnostic exams. Those who are prone to this condition are recommended to undergo regular screening and checkups. These simple actions could save a person's life.

Chapter 4 - Determining Anorexia Through Tests and Diagnostic Exams

The symptoms of Anorexia could serve as warnings to seek further testing. This is vital to ensure a good prognosis. The doctor may request the following tests, not only to establish the presence of Anorexia but also to determine the total wellbeing of the patient.

The tests may include the following:

1. Health history. Through interview, the patient would be asked about their personal profile, family health history, previous hospitalization and illnesses, vaccination, health habits and maintenance medicines if applicable. If the patient is a minor, the parents or guardian could answer on his or her behalf. However, the doctor will generally also want to have a separate interview with the patient, as parents or family culture, such as the drive for perfection, could be the cause of the illness. As anorexia is focused on food intake, the doctor will also ask about food-intake history and food preferences during the interview.

2. Physical Exam. There is the initial measurement of height and weight that will serve as the basis of reference for future checkups. The vital signs would also be taken and recorded. This would include temperature, pulse rate, blood pressure, and respiratory rate. A physical examination from head to toe would also be conducted. Checking of skin, nail, teeth, hair, plus examination of the heart, lungs, kidneys, and abdomen would also be conducted through palpation, percussion and auscultation.

3. Laboratory tests. A blood chemistry exam such as a complete blood count (CBC) would be requested. To check for electrolyte imbalances, more blood exams may be taken. Included in these are Potassium, Sodium, Magnesium, Calcium, and Phosphorous. A blood glucose exam could be taken to indicate if the patient is hypoglycemic or has low blood sugar because of the absence of food intake. Tests for the kidneys, liver and thyroid may be conducted also. The doctor may also ask for routine stool and urine analysis.

4. Psychological Evaluation. Since Anorexia is also a psychological concern, testing the psychological health of the individual is a must. The doctor will ask the patient to fill in a mental health assessment form to check for depression symptoms. A mental health provider would interview the patient regarding one's thoughts, feelings, eating habits and preferences.

To further determine the presence and severity of Anorexia, diagnostic examinations may also be required by the primary health care provider. This may include the following:

1. X-rays. To visualize the structure of the heart, lungs, skeletal system and the kidneys.

2. Electrocardiogram. This checks the electrical activity of the heart. Imbalances in the Potassium electrolyte would also be reflected here.

3. 2D Echo. Displays the cross section slice of the heart. The conditions of the heart's chambers, valves, and the major blood vessels would also be seen in this diagnostic exam.

4. Bone density testing. As the skeletal system could be affected, leading to brittle bones and fractures, bone health could be determined with this test.

Prioritize safety. Have an early screening and testing for Anorexia if you are at high risk for it. Doing so can prevent progression of the symptoms into serious health conditions. Likewise, if you think that a family member or friend is at risk of developing anorexia, encourage them to seek professional help and get these tests done. The sooner a prognosis is made, the sooner treatment can be started.

Chapter 5 - Focus of Treatment For Anorexia

Anorexia is a complex medical condition, which can be very challenging to treat. Why? The success of any treatment is usually dependent on the cooperation and participation of the patient. With anorexics, the acceptance that they are sick and in need of medical treatment is usually not present. Most of the time, they are in denial of the seriousness of their condition.

There are three priorities when treating Anorexia. First, address any serious health conditions as soon as possible. Second, get back to the healthy weight ideal for the body. Lastly, make sure that the patient does not go back to being anorexic through psychotherapy and family counseling.

Medical Management for Anorexia

The priority is to make sure that the patient is safe from any physical harm due to poor health. As discussed earlier, Anorexia can be potentially fatal if left untreated.

When the patient is not in critical danger, he or she can be treated as an outpatient. However, if the condition worsens, hospitalization is required. The doctor may order insertion of nasogastric tube for food to get inside the person. Intravenous fluid can be used to help hydrate the patient. If malnutrition is severe, total parenteral nutrition (TPN) would allow direct delivery of nutrients to the blood.

For patients who can cause harm to oneself or others, a 24-hour companion would be required to keep watch. Rehabilitation would also be required until such a time that the tendency to hurt oneself and others is gone. Suicidal tendencies are very high among anorexics.

Pharmacological therapy may include the following medicines: antidepressants, mood stabilizers and antipsychotics. Though these medicines have no direct effects on Anorexia, these drugs can treat the depression, which allows the patient to have a more positive outlook, leading to an increased appetite. Hormonal therapies, like those involving estrogen, are also recommended to help prevent bone problems such as osteoporosis and fractures. Supplements of vitamins, minerals and electrolytes are also administered to supply the body's requirements for these.

Nutritional Management For Anorexia

The next step in treating Anorexia is the reversal of the malnourished state through proper nutrition. It is expected that this focus of treatment may take several months or sometimes, years as the patient gradually tolerates intake of food without the psychological symptoms attached to it.

A nutritionist or dietician is the person responsible for educating the patient regarding proper nutrition and healthy eating. Together with the patient, the nutritionist plans and develops the meals appropriate for the patient's needs.

Here are some pointers to follow while caring for an anorexic at this time:

- Be a role model to the anorexic. Try to eat healthy. Avoid negative comments regarding people's weight or undernourished state.
- Encourage the anorexic to eat small, frequent meals. As the anorexic's stomach is used to a small amount of food only, a large intake of food may overwhelm the person and also the stomach. Five or six small meals a day is preferred over three large meals.

- Choose foods that are high in calories and protein. Even though the amount of food may be small, the calorie count and protein content helps to make up for that.
- As much as possible, meal times should be the happiest time. Avoid talking about problems and negative things during mealtimes.
- Increase fluid intake, not only of water but of other healthy drinks such as milk and fruit juice. However, refrain from drinking during meal times as this can cause feeling of fullness.
- Provide an ambience conducive for eating. The dishes should be attractive. The table should be clean and inviting. The temperature, both of the room and of the food, should just be just right. Remove distractions that may impede an enjoyable meal like television or gadgets. Make sure that the patient is comfortable.
- Provide ample time for the patient to eat. Do not rush meal times. It is not only about the quantity of food you are after but also the quality of mealtimes.
- Always have somebody with the client during and after meal times. This is to monitor that the person is eating the right amount of food and at the same time, prevents him or her from inducing vomiting or taking laxatives and diuretics after the meals.

Psychotherapy Approach for Anorexia

This therapy is very crucial to the anorexic for this will deal not only with the current condition of the client, but also the origin of the disorder. Once the very root has been taken care of, it's more likely that relapse will not occur. The goal is to develop a mental self-image that prevents the client from using Anorexia to gain self worth in the future.

The two most common psychotherapies for anorexics are:

1. Cognitive Behavioral Therapy (CBT). The main objective here is for the patient to realize how

destructive negative thoughts and perceptions are, as these can lead him or her to anorexia. There are many options under this therapy. One can go for the talk therapy – either with the patient or patient and their family. There are also relaxation strategies such as positive imaging, where the client is asked to visualize herself or himself, as healthy, confident and happy.

2. Family therapy. Family plays a major role in treating Anorexia. When one has a strong support system, one can move on to recovery much faster.

All three treatments are vital to the recovery of the anorexic. The complexity of this medical condition requires professional help. However, the anorexic's participation in the treatment and a strong support system will be the deciding factors of the success of the treatment.

Chapter 6 - Bidding Farewell to Anorexia

There is hope for anorexics. Anorexia has a cure. You can say goodbye to it for good. You do not have to suffer through life because of this eating disorder. Submission to the medical, nutritional and psychotherapy counseling are very important. However, the most crucial factor in totally beating this malady is YOU. Yes, you have the final control and decision making ability when it comes to Anorexia. Overcome poor self-image and be free from the need to lose weight by understanding that there is nothing wrong with you and your body.

Always uplift yourself by focusing on your strengths and not on your weaknesses. Do not be too hard on yourself. Nobody is perfect. Realize that perfection is not the key to happiness and success.

Stay active too. Activities and movement releases the brain chemicals serotonin and norepinephrine, giving you that overall good feeling. Spend time with family and close friends.

Enhance your spiritual life by participating in religious activities that you like. When one has inner peace, the need to impress others becomes insignificant.

The road to recovery from anorexia may not be easy, but it is a journey that you need to take if you currently suffer from the condition.

Conclusion

Thank you again for downloading this book!

I hope this book was able to help you learn more about anorexia!

The next step is to put this information to use, and begin working on improving your condition!

While it's not easy to overcome anorexia, it's something that you are definitely capable of achieving. Know that others around you are there for you, even though you might not feel like asking for help. Follow the advice in this book, and begin working towards living a life free of anorexia!

Finally, if you enjoyed this book, please take the time to share your thoughts and post a review on Amazon. It'd be greatly appreciated!

Thank you and good luck!

www.ingramcontent.com/pod-product-compliance
Lightning Source LLC
LaVergne TN
LVHW021749060526
838200LV00052B/3556